Diabetic Diet Cookbook

2021

50 Tasty and Affordable Diabetic Diet Recipes for our everyday meals

Roseann Smith

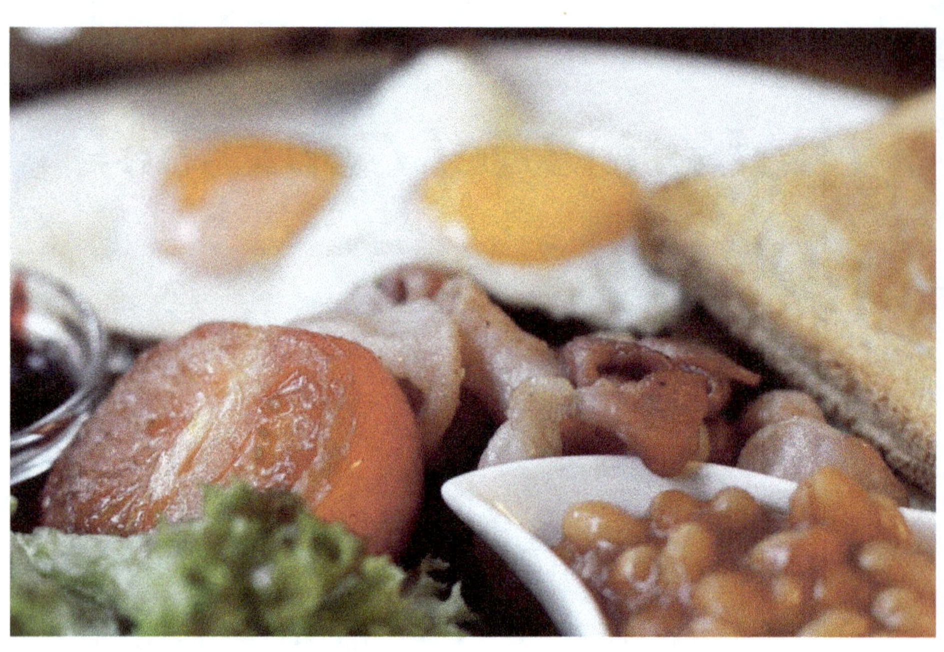

Disclaimer Notice:

Please note the information contained within this document is for educational and entertainment purposes only. All effort has been executed to present accurate, up to date, and reliable, complete information. No warranties of any kind are declared or implied. Readers acknowledge that the author is not engaging in the rendering of legal, financial, medical or professional advice. The content within this book has been derived from various sources. Please consult a licensed professional before attempting any techniques outlined in this book.

By reading this document, the reader agrees that under no circumstances is the author responsible for any losses, direct or indirect, which are incurred as a result of the use of information contained within this document, including, but not limited to, — errors, omissions, or inaccuracies.

Table of Contents

Vegetable Frittata

Servings: 2

Cooking Time: 20 Minutes

Ingredients:

- 1 cup mushrooms, sliced
- 4 eggs, beaten lightly
- 2 tablespoons onion, chopped
- ½ cup broccoli, chopped
- ¼ cup cheddar cheese, shredded, low-fat
- What you will need from the store cupboard:
- 2 tablespoons green pepper, chopped
- Dash of pepper
- 1/8 teaspoon of salt
- Cooking spray

Directions:

1. Bring together all the ingredients in your bowl.
2. Coat your baking dish with cooking spray and pour everything into it.
3. Bake for 20 minutes and serve immediately.

Nutrition Info: Calories 230, Carbohydrates 6g, Fiber 1g, Sugar 0.2g, Cholesterol 386mg, Total Fat 14g, Protein 20g

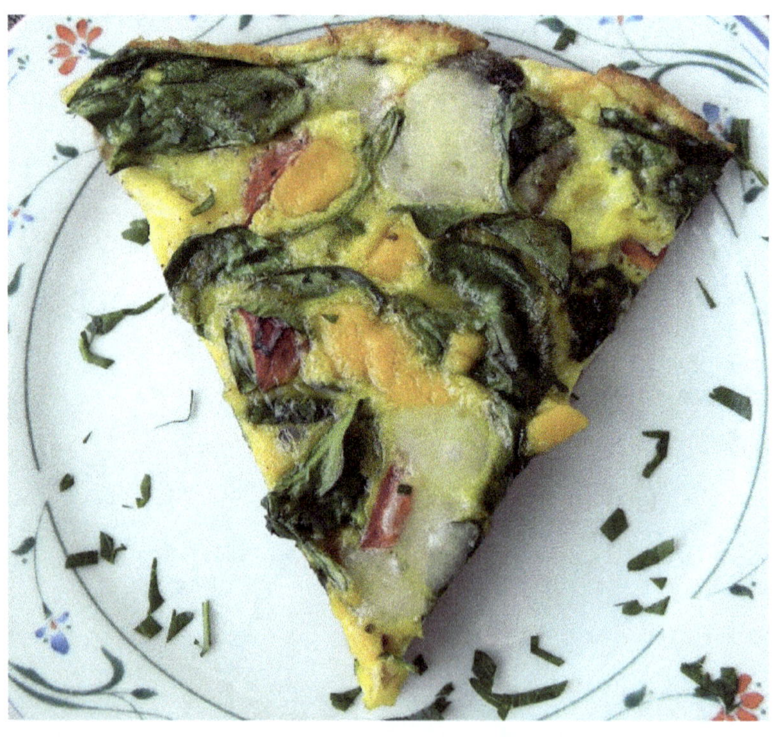

Egg-veggie Scramble

Servings: 2

Cooking Time: 3 Minutes

Ingredients:

- ¼ tsp salt
- 1 tbsp unsalted butter
- 1/8 tsp ground black pepper
- 3 eggs, beaten
- 4 oz spinach

Directions:

1. Bring out a frying pan, put it over medium heat, add butter and when it melts, add spinach and cook for 5 minutes until leaves have wilted.

2. Then pour in eggs, season with salt and black pepper, and cook for 3 minutes until eggs have scramble to the desired level.

Nutrition Info: 90 Cal 7 g Fats 5.6 g Protein; 0.7 g Net Carb 0.6 g Fiber

Apple Omelet

Servings: 3

Cooking Time: 10 Minutes

Ingredients:

- 4 teaspoons olive oil, divided
- 2 small green apples, cored and sliced thinly
- ¼ teaspoon ground cinnamon
- Pinch of ground cloves
- Pinch of ground nutmeg
- 4 large eggs
- ¼ teaspoon organic vanilla extract
- Pinch of salt

Directions:

1. over medium-low heat in frying pan, heat 1 teaspoon
2. Place the apple slices and sprinkle with spices.
3. Cook for about 4-5 minutes, flipping once halfway through.
4. Meanwhile, in a bowl, add the eggs, vanilla extract and salt and beat until fluffy.
5. Add the remaining oil in the pan and let it heat completely.
6. Place the egg mixture over apple slices evenly and cook for about 3-5 minutes or until desired doneness.
7. Carefully, turn the pan over a serving plate and immediately, fold the omelet.
8. Serve immediately.

Nutrition Info: Calories 228 Total Fat 13.2 g Saturated Fat 3 g Cholesterol 248 mg Total Carbs 21.3 g Sugar 16.1 g Fiber 3.8 g Sodium 145 mg Potassium 251 mg Protein 8.8 g

Mix Veggie Fritters

Servings: 2

Cooking Time: 3 Minutes

Ingredients:

- ½ tsp nutritional yeast
- 1 oz chopped broccoli
- 1 zucchini, grated, squeezed
- 2 eggs
- 2 tbsp almond flour

Directions:

1. Wrap grated zucchini in a cheesecloth, twist it well to remove excess moisture, and then Put zucchini in a bowl.
2. Add remaining ingredients, except for oil, and then whisk well until combined.
3. Bring out a skillet pan, put it over medium heat, add oil and when hot, drop zucchini mixture in four portions, shape them into flat

patties and cook for 4 minutes per side until thoroughly cooked.

Nutrition Info: 191 Cal 16.6 g Fats 9.6 g Protein 0.8 g Net Carb 0.2 g Fiber

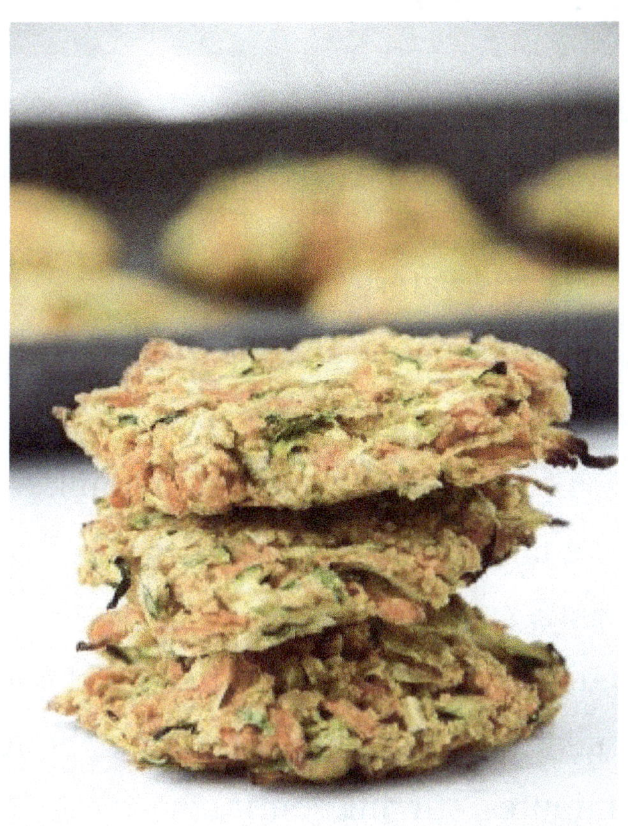

Millet Porridge

Servings: 4

Cooking Time: 25 Minutes

Ingredients:

- 1 cup millet, rinsed and drained
- Pinch of salt
- 3 cups water
- 2 tablespoons almonds, chopped finely
- 6-8 drops liquid stevia
- 1 cup unsweetened almond milk
- 2 tablespoons fresh blueberries

Directions:

1. In a nonstick pan, add the millet over medium-low heat and cook for about 3 minutes, stirring continuously.
2. Add the salt and water and stir to combine
3. Increase the heat to medium and bring to a boil.

4.   Cook for about 15 minutes.

5.   Stir in the almonds, stevia and almond milk and cook for 5 minutes.

6.   Top with the blueberries and serve.

Nutrition Info: Calories 219 Total Fat 4.5 g Saturated Fat 0.6 g Cholesterol 0 mg Total Carbs 38.2 g Sugar 0.6 g Fiber 5 g Sodium 92 mg Potassium 1721 mg Protein 6.4 g

Steel-cut Oatmeal Bowl With Fruit And Nuts

Servings: 4

Cooking Time: 20 Minutes

Ingredients:

- 1 cup steel-cut oats
- 2 cups almond milk
- ¾ cup water
- 1 teaspoon ground cinnamon
- ¼ teaspoon salt
- 2 cups chopped fresh fruit, such as blueberries, strawberries, raspberries, or peaches
- 1/2 cup chopped walnuts
- ¼ cup chia seeds

Directions:

1. In a medium saucepan over medium-high heat, combine the oats, almond milk, water, cinnamon, and salt. Bring to a boil, reduce the heat to low, and simmer for 15 to 20 minutes, until the oats are softened and thickened.

2. Top each bowl with 1/2 cup of fresh fruit, 2 tablespoons of walnuts, and 1 tablespoon of chia seeds before serving.

Nutrition Info: Calories: 288; Total fat: 11g; Saturated fat: 1g; Protein: 10g; Carbs: 38g; Sugar: 7g; Fiber: 10g; Cholesterol: 0mg; Sodium: 329mg

Salty Macadamia Chocolate Smoothie

Servings: 1

Cooking Time: Nil

Ingredients:

- 2 tablespoons macadamia nuts, salted
- 1/3 cup chocolate whey protein powder, low carb
- 1 cup almond milk, unsweetened

Directions:

1. Add the listed ingredients to your blender and blend until you have a smooth mixture
2. Chill and enjoy it!

Nutrition Info: Calories: 165; Fat: 2g; Carbohydrates: 1g; Protein: 12g

Tofu & Zucchini Muffins

Servings: 6

Cooking Time: 40 Minutes

Ingredients:

- 12 ounces extra-firm silken tofu, drained and pressed
- ¾ cup unsweetened soy milk
- 2 tablespoons canola oil
- 1 tablespoon apple cider vinegar
- 1 cup whole-wheat pastry flour
- ½ cup chickpea flour
- 1 teaspoon baking powder
- ½ teaspoon baking soda
- 1 teaspoon smoked paprika
- 1 teaspoon onion powder
- 1 teaspoon salt
- ½ cup zucchini, chopped
- ¼ cup fresh chives, minced

Directions:

1. Preheat your oven to 400°F.
2. Line a 12-cup muffin tin with paper liners.
3. In a bowl, place tofu and with a fork, mash until smooth.
4. In the bowl of tofu, add almond milk, oil, and vinegar, and mix until slightly smooth.
5. In a separate large bowl, add flours, baking powder, baking soda, spices, and salt, and mix well.
6. Transfer the mixture into muffin cups evenly.
7. Bake for approximately 35–40 minutes or until a toothpick inserted in the center comes out clean.
8. Remove the muffin tin from oven and place onto a wire rack to cool for about 10 minutes.
9. Carefully invert the muffins onto a platter and serve warm.

Nutrition Info: Calories 237 Total Fat 9 g Saturated Fat 1 g Cholesterol 0 mg Sodium 520 mg Total Carbs 2293.3 g Fiber 5.9 g Sugar 3.7 g Protein 11.1 g

Savory Keto Pancake

Servings: 2

Cooking Time: 2 Minutes

Ingredients:

- ¼ cup almond flour
- 1 ½ tbsp unsalted butter
- 2 eggs
- 2 oz cream cheese, softened

Directions:

1. Bring out a bowl, crack eggs in it, whisk well until fluffy, and then whisk in flour and cream cheese until well combined.

2. Bring out a skillet pan, put it over medium heat, add butter and when it melts, drop pancake batter in four sections, spread it evenly, and cook for 2 minutes per side until brown.

Nutrition Info: 166.8 Cal 15 g Fats 5.8 g Protein 1.8 g Net Car 0.8 g Fiber

Sweet Potato Waffles

Servings: 2

Cooking Time: 20 Minutes

Ingredients:

- 1 medium sweet potato, peeled, grated and squeezed
- 1 teaspoon fresh thyme, minced
- 1 teaspoon fresh rosemary, minced
- 1/8 teaspoon red pepper flakes, crushed
- Salt and ground black pepper, as required

Directions:

1. Preheat the waffle iron and then grease it.
2. In a large bowl, add all ingredients and mix till well combined.
3. Place half of the sweet potato mixture into preheated waffle iron and cook for about 8-10 minutes or until golden brown.
4. Repeat with the remaining mixture.
5. Serve warm.

Nutrition Info: Calories 72 Total Fat 0.3 g Saturated Fat 0.1 g Cholesterol 0 mg Total Carbs 16.3 g Sugar 4.9 g Fiber 3 g Sodium 28 mg Potassium 369 mg Protein 1.6 g

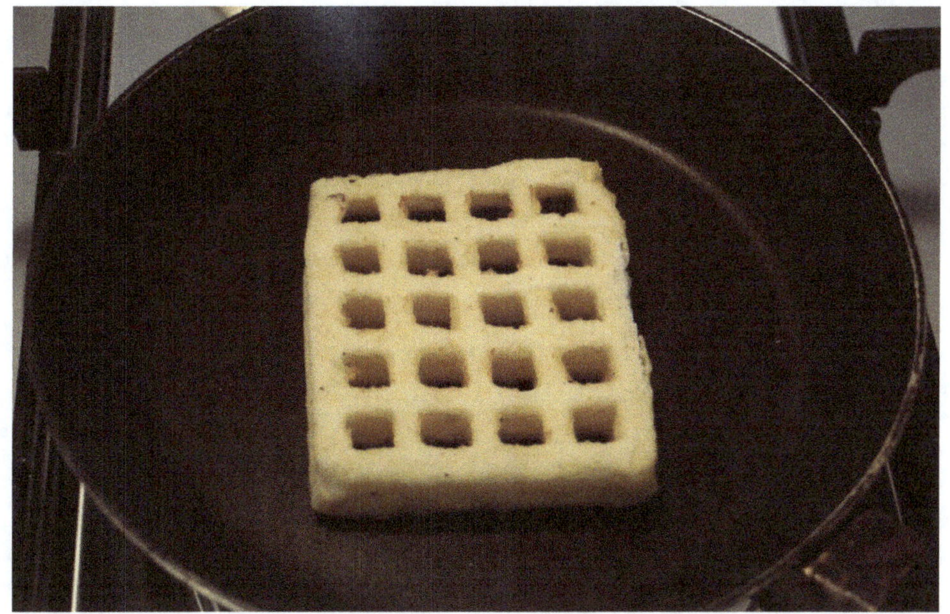

Buckwheat Porridge

Servings: 2

Cooking Time: 15 Minutes

Ingredients:

- 1½ cups water
- 1 cup buckwheat groats, rinsed
- ¾ teaspoon vanilla extract
- ½ teaspoon ground cinnamon
- ¼ teaspoon salt
- 2 tablespoons maple syrup
- 1 ripe banana, peeled and mashed
- 1½ cups unsweetened soy milk
- 1 tablespoon peanut butter
- 1/3 cup fresh strawberries, hulled and chopped

Directions:

1. Place the water, buckwheat, vanilla extract, cinnamon, and salt in a pan and bring to a boil.
2. Now, adjust the heat to medium-low and simmer for about 6 minutes, stirring occasionally.
3. Stir in maple syrup, banana, and soy milk, and simmer, covered for about 6 minutes.
4. Remove the pan of porridge from heat and stir in peanut butter.
5. Serve warm with the topping of strawberry pieces.

Nutrition Info: Calories 453 Total Fat 9.4 g Saturated Fat 1.7 g Cholesterol 0 mg Sodium 374 mg Total Carbs 82.8 g Fiber 9.4 g Sugar 28.8 g Protein 16.2 g

Breakfast Sandwich

Servings: 2

Cooking Time: 0 Minutes

Ingredients:

- 2 oz/60g cheddar cheese
- 1/6 oz/30g smoked ham
- 2 tbsp butter
- 4 eggs

Directions:

1. Fry all the eggs and sprinkle the pepper and salt on them.
2. Place an egg down as the sandwich base. Top with the ham and cheese and a drop or two of Tabasco.
3. Place the other egg on top and enjoy.

Nutrition Info: 600 cal.50g fat 12g protein 7g carbs.

Berry-oat Breakfast Bars

7Servings: 12

Cooking Time: 25 Minutes

Ingredients:

- 2 cups fresh raspberries or blueberries
- 2 tablespoons sugar
- 2 tablespoons freshly squeezed lemon juice
- 1 tablespoon cornstarch
- 11/2 cups rolled oats
- 1/2 cup whole-wheat flour
- 1/2 cup walnuts
- ¼ cup chia seeds
- ¼ cup extra-virgin olive oil
- ¼ cup honey
- 1 large egg

Directions:

1. Preheat the oven to 350F.

2. In a small saucepan over medium heat, stir together the berries, sugar, lemon juice, and cornstarch. Bring to a simmer. Reduce the heat and simmer for 2 to 3 minutes, until the mixture thickens.

3. In a food processor or high-speed blender, combine the oats, flour, walnuts, and chia seeds. Process until powdered. Add the olive oil, honey, and egg. Pulse a few more times, until well combined. Press half of the mixture into a 9-inch square baking dish.

4. Spread the berry filling over the oat mixture. Add the remaining oat mixture on top of the berries. Bake for 25 minutes, until browned.

5. Let cool completely, cut into 12 pieces, and serve. Store in a covered container for up to 5 days.

Nutrition Info: Calories: 201; Total fat: 10g; Saturated fat: 1g; Protein: 5g; Carbs: 26g; Sugar: 9g; Fiber: 5g; Cholesterol: 16mg; Sodium: 8mg 30 MINUTES OR LESS • NUT FREE • VEGETARIAN

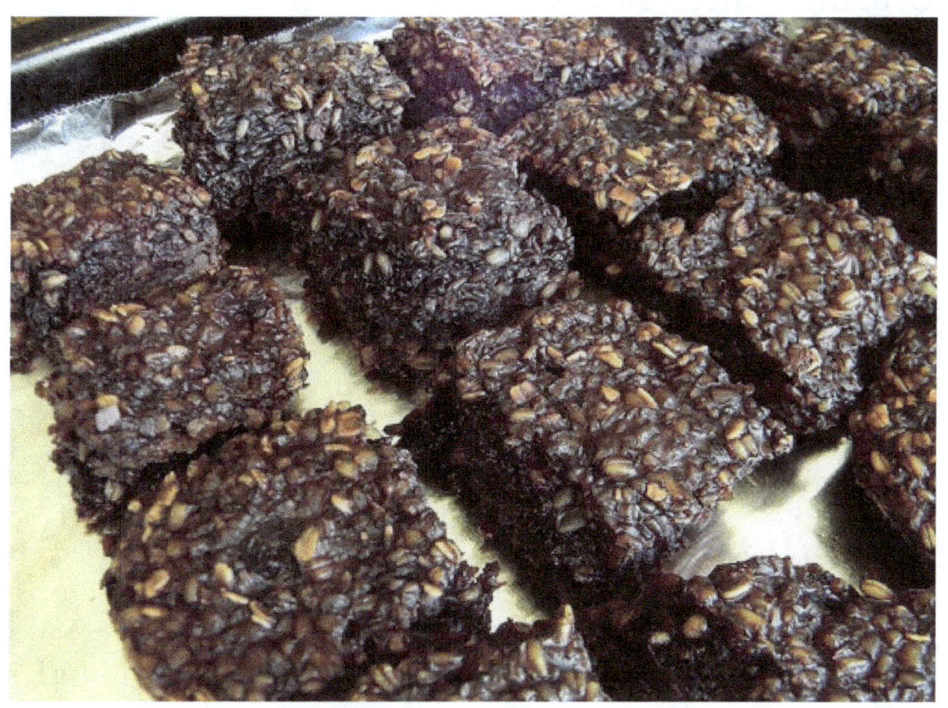

Eggplant Omelet

Servings: 2

Cooking Time: 5 Minutes

Ingredients:

- 1 large eggplant
- 1 tbsp coconut oil, melted
- 1 tsp unsalted butter
- 2 eggs
- 2 tbsp chopped green onions

Directions:

1. Set the grill and let it preheat at the high setting.

2. In the meantime, Prepare the eggplant, and for this, cut two slices from eggplant, about 1-inch thick, and reserve the remaining eggplant for later use.

3. Brush slices of eggplant with oil, season with salt on both sides, then Put the slices on grill and cook for 3 to 4 minutes per side.

4. Move grilled eggplant to a cutting board, let it cool for 5 minutes and then make a home in the center of each slice by using a cookie cutter.

5. Bring out a frying pan, put it over medium heat, add butter and when it melts, add eggplant slices in it and crack an egg into its each hole.

6. Let the eggs cook, then carefully flip the eggplant slice and continue cooking for 3 minutes until the egg has thoroughly cooked

7. Season egg with salt and black pepper, move them to a plate, then garnish with green onions and serve.

Nutrition Info: 184 Cal 14.1 g Fats 7.8 g Protein 3 g Net Carb 3.5 g Fiber

Breakfast Muffins

Servings: 1

Cooking Time: 5 Minutes

Ingredients:

- 1 medium egg
- ¼ cup heavy cream
- 1 slice cooked bacon (cured, pan-fried, cooked)
- 1 oz cheddar cheese
- Salt and black pepper (to taste)

Directions:

1. Preheat the oven to 350°F.
2. In a bowl, mix the eggs with the cream, salt and pepper.
3. Spread into muffin tins and fill the cups half full.
4. Place 1 slice of bacon into each muffin hole and half ounce of cheese on top of each muffin.

5. Bake for around 15-20 minutes or until slightly browned.

6. Add another ½ oz of cheese onto each muffin and broil until the cheese is slightly browned. Serve!

Nutrition Info: 150 cal 11g fat 7g protein 2g carbs

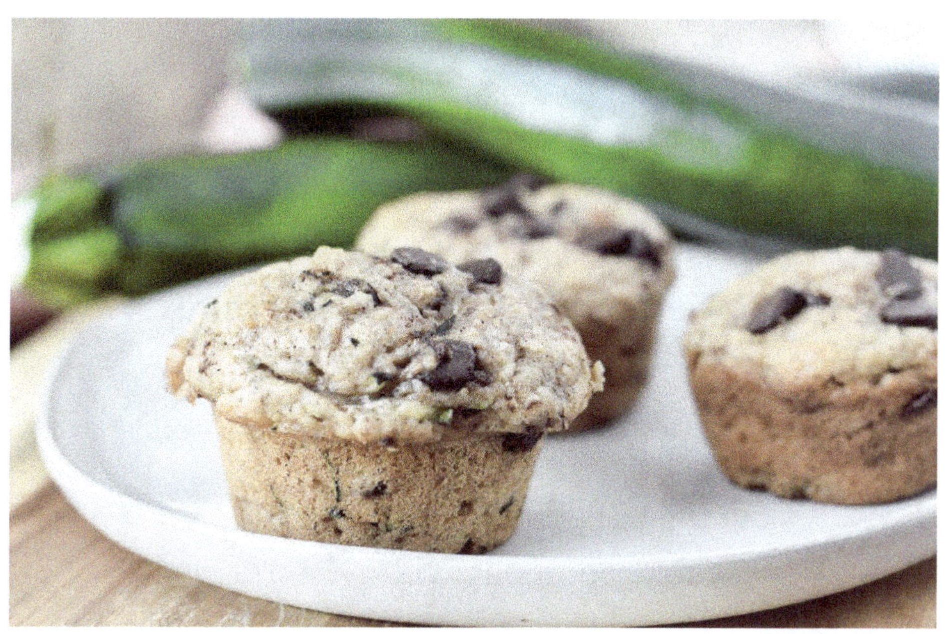

Stuffed Chicken Breasts Greek-style

Servings: 4

Cooking Time: 20 Minutes

Ingredients:

- 4 oz. chicken breasts, skinless and boneless
- ¼ cup onion, minced
- 4 artichoke hearts, minced
- 1 teaspoon oregano, crushed
- 4 lemon slices
- What you will need from the store cupboard:
- 1 cup canned chicken broth, fat-free
- 1-1/2 lemon juice
- 1 tablespoon olive oil
- 2 teaspoons of cornstarch
- Ground pepper
- Salt, optional

Directions:

1. Take out all the fat from the chicken. Wash and pat dry.
2. Season your chicken with pepper and salt.
3. Pound the chicken to make it flat and thin.
4. Bring together the oregano, onion, and artichoke hearts.
5. Now spoon equal amounts of the mix at the center of your chicken.
6. Roll up the log and secure using a skewer or toothpick.
7. Heat oil in your skillet over medium temperature.
8. Add the chicken. Brown all sides evenly.
9. Pour the lemon juice and broth.
10. Add lemon slices on top of the chicken. Simmer covered for 10 minutes.
11. Transfer to a platter. Remove the skewers or toothpick.
12. Mix cornstarch with a fork.
13. Transfer to skillet and stir over high temperature.

14. Put lemon sauce on the chicken.

Nutrition Info: Calories 224, Carbohydrates 8g, Fiber 1g, Cholesterol 82mg, Total Fat 5g, Protein 21g, Sodium 339mg

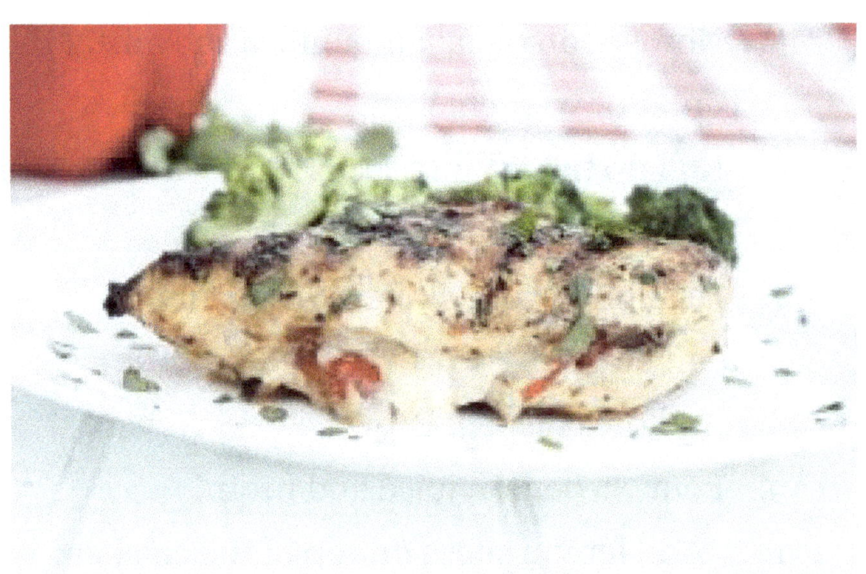

Shredded Beef

Servings: 2

Cooking Time: 35 Minutes

Ingredients:

- 1.5lb lean steak
- 1 cup low sodium gravy
- 2tbsp mixed spices

Directions:

1. Mix all the ingredients in your Instant Pot.
2. Cook on Stew for 35 minutes.
3. Release the pressure naturally.
4. Shred the beef.

Nutrition Info: Calories: 200 Carbs: 2 Sugar: 0 Fat: 5 Protein: 48 GL: 1

Classic Mini Meatloaf

Servings: 6

Cooking Time: 25 Minutes

Ingredients:

- 1 pound 80/20 ground beef
- ¼ medium yellow onion, peeled and diced
- ½ medium green bell pepper, seeded and diced
- 1 large egg
- 3 tablespoons blanched finely ground almond flour
- 1 tablespoon Worcestershire sauce
- ½ teaspoon garlic powder
- 1 teaspoon dried parsley
- 2 tablespoons tomato paste
- ¼ cup water
- 1 tablespoon powdered erythritol

Directions:

1. In a large bowl, combine ground beef, onion, pepper, egg, and almond flour. Pour in the Worcestershire sauce and add the garlic powder and parsley to the bowl. Mix until fully combined.

2. Divide the mixture into two and place into two (4") loaf baking pans.

3. In a small bowl, mix the tomato paste, water, and erythritol. Spoon half the mixture over each loaf.

4. Working in batches if necessary, place loaf pans into the air fryer basket.

5. Adjust the temperature to 350°F and set the timer for 25 minutes or until internal temperature is 180°F.

6. Serve warm.

Nutrition Info: Calories: 170 Protein: 14.9 G Fiber: 0.9 G Net Carbohydrates: 2.6 G Sugar Alcohol: 1.5 G Fat: 9.4 G Sodium: 85 Mg Carbohydrates: 5.0 G Sugar: 1.5 G

Skirt Steak With Asian Peanut Sauce

Servings: 4

Cooking Time: 15 Minutes

Ingredients:

- ⅓ cup light coconut milk
- 1 teaspoon curry powder
- 1 teaspoon coriander powder
- 1 teaspoon reduced-sodium soy sauce
- 1¼ pound skirt steak
- Cooking spray
- ½ cup Asian Peanut Sauce

Directions:

1. In a large bowl, whisk together the coconut milk, curry powder, coriander powder, and soy sauce. Add the steak and turn to coat. Cover the bowl and refrigerate for at least 30 minutes and no longer than 24 hours.

2. Preheat the barbecue or coat a grill pan with cooking spray and place the steak over medium-high heat. Grill the meat until it reaches an internal temperature of 145°F, about 3 minutes per side. Remove the steak from the grill and let it rest for 5 minutes. Slice the steak into 5-ounce pieces and serve each with 2 tablespoons of the Asian Peanut Sauce.

3. REFRIGERATE: Store the cooled steak in a reseal able container for up to 1 week. Reheat each piece in the microwave for 1 minute.

Nutrition Info: Calories: 361 Fat: 22g Saturated Fat: 7g Protein: 36g Total Carbs: 8g Fiber: 2g Sodium: 349mg

Roasted Pork Loin With Grainy Mustard Sauce

Servings: 8

Cooking Time: 70 Minutes

Ingredients:

- 1 (2-pound) boneless pork loin roast
- Sea salt
- Freshly ground black pepper
- 3 tablespoons olive oil
- 1½ cups heavy (whipping) cream
- 3 tablespoons grainy mustard, such as Pommery

Directions:

1. Preheat the oven to 375°F.
2. Season the pork roast all over with sea salt and pepper.
3. Place a large skillet over medium-high heat and add the olive oil.

4. Brown the roast on all sides in the skillet, about 6 minutes in total, and place the roast in a baking dish.

5. Roast until a meat thermometer inserted in the thickest part of the roast reads 155°F, about 1 hour.

6. When there is approximately 15 minutes of roasting time left, place a small saucepan over medium heat and add the heavy cream and mustard.

7. Stir the sauce until it simmers, then reduce the heat to low. Simmer the sauce until it is very rich and thick, about 5 minutes. Remove the pan from the heat and set aside.

8. Let the pork rest for 10 minutes before slicing and serve with the sauce.

Nutrition Info: Calories 368 Fat: 29g Protein: 25g Carbs: 2g Fiber: 0g Net Carbs: 2g Fat 70%/Protein 25%/Carbs 5%

Meatballs In Tomato Gravy

Servings: 6

Cooking Time: 30 Minutes

Ingredients:

- For Meatballs:
- 1 pound lean ground lamb
- 1 tablespoon homemade tomato paste
- ¼ cup fresh cilantro leaves, chopped
- 1 small onion, chopped finely
- 2 garlic cloves, minced
- ½ teaspoon ground cumin
- 1/8 teaspoon salt
- Ground black pepper, as required
- For Tomato Gravy:
- 3 tablespoons olive oil, divided
- 2 medium onions, chopped finely
- 2 garlic cloves, minced
- ½ tablespoon fresh ginger, minced

- 1 teaspoon dried thyme, crushed
- 1 teaspoon dried oregano, crushed
- 3 large tomatoes, chopped finely
- Ground black pepper, as required
- 1½ cups warm low-sodium chicken broth

Directions:

1. For meatballs: in a large bowl, add all the ingredients and mix until well combined.
2. Make small equal-sized balls from mixture and set aside.
3. For gravy: in a large pan, heat 1 tablespoon of oil over medium heat.
4. Add the meatballs and cook for about 4-5 minutes or until lightly browned from all sides.
5. With a slotted spoon, transfer the meatballs onto a plate.
6. In the same pan, heat the remaining oil over medium heat and sauté the onion for about 8-10 minutes.
7. Add the garlic, ginger and herbs and sauté for about 1 minute.

8. Add the tomatoes and cook for about 3-4 minutes, crushing with the back of spoon.

9. Add the warm broth and bring to a boil.

10. Carefully, place the meatballs and cook for 5 minutes, without stirring.

11. Now, reduce the heat to low and cook partially covered for about 15-20 minutes, stirring gently 2-3 times.

12. Serve hot.

13. Meal Prep Tip: Transfer the meatballs mixture into a large bowl and set aside to cool. Divide the mixture into 6 containers evenly. Cover the containers and refrigerate for 1-2 days. Reheat in the microwave before serving.

Nutrition Info: Calories 248 Total Fat 12.9 g Saturated Fat 3 g Cholesterol 68 mg Total Carbs 10 g Sugar 4.8 g Fiber 2.5 g Sodium 138 mg Potassium 591 mg Protein 23.4 g

Garlic-braised Short Rib

Servings: 4

Cooking Time: 2 Hours, 20 Minutes

Ingredients:

- 4 (4-ounce) beef short ribs
- Sea salt
- Freshly ground black pepper
- 1 tablespoon olive oil
- 2 teaspoons minced garlic
- ½ cup dry red wine
- 3 cups Rich Beef Stock (here)

Directions:

1. Preheat the oven to 325°F.
2. Season the beef ribs on all sides with salt and pepper.
3. Place a deep ovenproof skillet over medium-high heat and add the olive oil.

4.   Sear the ribs on all sides until browned, about 6 minutes in total. Transfer the ribs to a plate.

5.   Add the garlic to the skillet and sauté until translucent, about 3 minutes.

6.   Whisk in the red wine to deglaze the pan. Be sure to scrape all the browned bits from the meat from the bottom of the pan. Simmer the wine until it is slightly reduced, about 2 minutes.

7.   Add the beef stock, ribs, and any accumulated juices on the plate back to the skillet and bring the liquid to a boil.

8.   Cover the skillet and place it in the oven to braise the ribs until the meat is fall-off-the-bone tender, about 2 hours.

9.   Serve the ribs with a spoonful of the cooking liquid drizzled over each serving.

Nutrition Info: Calories: 481 Fat: 38g Protein: 29g Carbs: 5g Fiber: 3g Net Carbs: 2g Fat 70%/Protein 25%/Carbs 5%

Pulled Pork

Servings: 8

Cooking Time: 2½ Hours

Ingredients:

- 2 tablespoons chili powder
- 1 teaspoon garlic powder
- ½ teaspoon onion powder
- ½ teaspoon ground black pepper
- ½ teaspoon cumin

Directions:

1. (4-pound) pork shoulder
2. In a small bowl, mix chili powder, garlic powder, onion powder, pepper, and cumin. Rub the spice mixture over the pork shoulder, patting it into the skin. Place pork shoulder into the air fryer basket.
3. Adjust the temperature to 350°F and set the timer for 150 minutes.

4. Pork skin will be crispy and meat easily shredded with two forks when done. The internal temperature should be at least 145°F.

Nutrition Info: Calories: 537 Protein: 42.6 G Fiber: 0.8 G Net Carbohydrates: 0.7 G Fat: 35.5 G Sodium: 180 Mg Carbohydrates: 1.5 G Sugar: 0.2 G

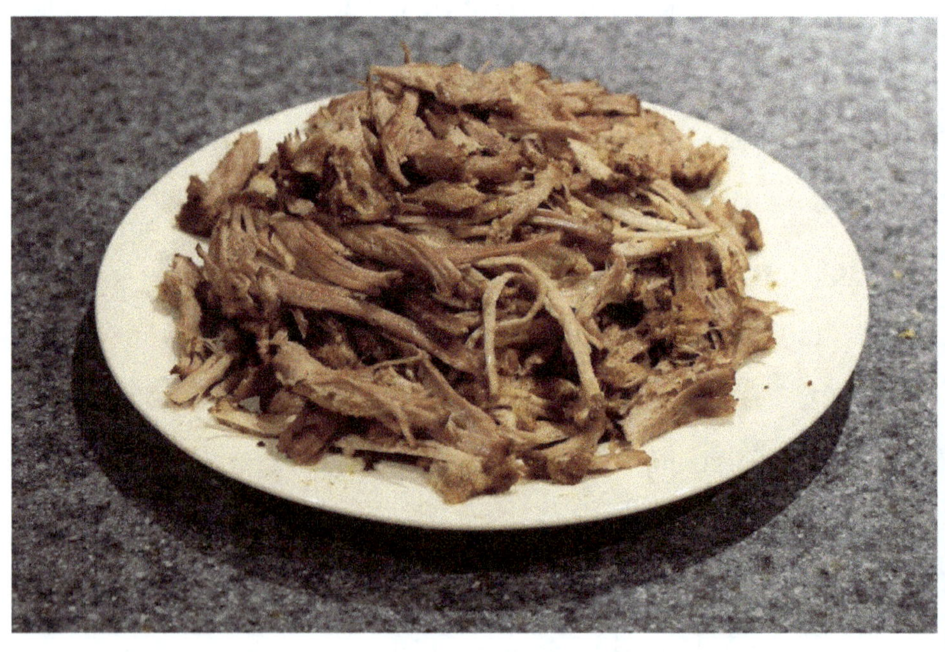

Rosemary-garlic Lamb Racks

Servings: 4

Cooking Time: 25 Minutes

Ingredients:

- 4 tablespoons extra-virgin olive oil
- 2 tablespoons finely chopped fresh rosemary
- 2 teaspoons minced garlic
- Pinch sea salt
- 2 (1-pound) racks French-cut lamb chops (8 bones each)

Directions:

1. In a small bowl, whisk together the olive oil, rosemary, garlic, and salt.
2. Place the racks in a sealable freezer bag and pour the olive oil mixture into the bag. Massage the meat through the bag so it is coated with the marinade. Press the air out of the bag and seal it.

3. Marinate the lamb racks in the refrigerator for 1 to 2 hours.

4. Preheat the oven to 450°F.

5. Place a large ovenproof skillet over medium-high heat. Take the lamb racks out of the bag and sear them in the skillet on all sides, about 5 minutes in total.

6. Arrange the racks upright in the skillet, with the bones interlaced, and roast them in the oven until they reach your desired doneness, about 20 minutes for medium-rare or until the internal temperature reaches 125°F.

7. Let the lamb rest for 10 minutes and then cut the racks into chops.

8. Serve 4 chops per person.

Nutrition Info: Calories: 354 Fat: 30g Protein: 21g Carbs: 0g Fiber: 0g Net Carbs: 0g Fat 70%/Protein 30%/Carbs 0%

Pork Chops In Peach Glaze

Servings: 2

Cooking Time: 16 Minutes

Ingredients:

- 2 (6-ounce) boneless pork chops, trimmed
- Sea Salt and ground black pepper, as required
- ½ of ripe yellow peach, peeled, pitted and chopped
- 1 tablespoon olive oil
- 2 tablespoons shallot, minced
- 2 tablespoons garlic, minced
- 2 tablespoons fresh ginger, minced
- 4-6 drops liquid stevia
- 1 tablespoon balsamic vinegar
- ¼ teaspoon red pepper flakes, crushed
- ¼ cup filtered water

Directions:

1. Season the pork chops with sea salt and black pepper generously.
2. In a blender, add the peach pieces and pulse until a puree forms.
3. Reserve the remaining peach pieces.
4. In a skillet, heat the oil over medium heat and sauté the shallots for about 1-2 minutes.
5. Add the garlic and ginger and sauté for about 1 minute.
6. Stir in the remaining ingredients and bring to a boil.
7. Now, reduce the heat to medium-low and simmer for about 4-5 minutes or until a sticky glaze forms.
8. Remove from the heat and reserve 1/3 of the glaze and set aside.
9. Coat the chops with remaining glaze.
10. Heat a nonstick skillet over medium-high heat and sear the chops for about 4 minutes per side.

11. Transfer the chops onto a plate and coat with the remaining glaze evenly.

12. Serve immediately.

13. Meal Prep Tip: Transfer the pork chops into a large bowl and set aside to cool. Divide the chops into 2 containers evenly. Cover the containers and refrigerate for 1-2 days. Reheat in the microwave before serving.

Nutrition Info: Calories 359 Total Fat 13.5 g Saturated Fat 3.2 g Cholesterol 124 mg Total Carbs 12 g Sugar 3.8 g Fiber 1.5 g Sodium 102 mg Potassium 938 mg Protein 46.2 g

Pan Grilled Steak

Servings: 4

Cooking Time: 16 Minutes

Ingredients:

- 8 medium garlic cloves, crushed
- 1 (2-inch) piece fresh ginger, sliced thinly
- ¼ cup olive oil
- Salt and ground black pepper, as required
- 1½ pounds flank steak, trimmed

Directions:

1. In a large sealable bag, mix together all ingredients except steak.
2. Add the steak and coat with marinade generously.
3. Seal the bag and refrigerate to marinate for about 24 hours.
4. Remove from refrigerator and keep in room temperature for about 15 minutes.
5. Discard the excess marinade from steak.

6.   Heat a lightly greased grill pan over medium-high heat and cook the steak for about 6-8 minutes per side.

7.   Remove from grill pan and set aside for about 10 minutes before slicing.

8.   With a sharp knife cut into desired slices and serve.

9.   Meal Prep Tip: Transfer the teak slices onto a wire rack to cool completely. With foil pieces, wrap the steak slices and refrigerate for about 1-2 days. Reheat in the microwave before serving.

Nutrition Info: Calories 447 Total Fat 26.8 g Saturated Fat 7.7 g Cholesterol 94 mg Total Carbs 2.1g Sugar 0.1 g Fiber 0.2 g Sodium 96 mg Potassium 601 mg Protein 47.7 g

Air Fryer Beef Empanadas

Servings: 3

Cooking Time: 20 Minutes

Ingredients:

- 8 Goya empanada discs, defrosted
- 1 cup picadillo
- 1 egg white, blended
- 1 tsp. water
- Cooking spray

Directions:

1. Set air fryer at 325 degrees F.
2. Apply a cooking spray to the basket.
3. Place 2 tbsps. of picadillo to each disc space. Fold in half and secure using a fork. Do the same for all the dough.

4.   Mix water and egg whites. Sprinkle to empanadas top.

5.   Set 3 of them in your air fryer and allow to bake for minutes. Set aside and do the same for the remaining empanadas.

Nutrition   Info: Calories:183   kcal   Carbs: 22g Protein:11 g Fat:5g

Thyme And Apple Chicken

Servings: 4

Cooking Time: 20 Minutes

Ingredients:

- 2 chicken breasts, boneless and skinless
- 1 teaspoon thyme leaves, crushed
- 1 green apple, cored, sliced thin
- 1 shallot, minced
- Thyme sprigs for garnishing
- What you will need from the store cupboard:
- ¼ cup balsamic vinegar
- Salt and pepper to taste
- Cooking spray

Directions:

1. Preheat your oven to 350 °F. Apply cooking spray on your baking dish lightly.

2. Rinse the chicken breasts. Use paper towels to pat dry.

3. Sprinkle salt and pepper on the breasts.

4. Place on your baking dish in a single layer.

5. Keep apple slices around and over the chicken.

6. Sprinkle thyme leaves and shallot.

7. Pour the balsamic vinegar.

8. Bake for 10 minutes.

9. Keep the cooked chicken breasts on a platter.

10. Spoon the cooking juice and apples on top.

11. You can garnish with thyme.

Nutrition Info: Calories 163, Carbohydrates 9g, Fiber 1g, Cholesterol 66mg, Total Fat 2g, Protein 27g, Sodium 78mg

Spiced Leg Of Lamb

Servings: 6

Cooking Time: 1 Hour 40 Minutes

Ingredients:

- For Marinade:
- 2/3 cup fat-free plain Greek yogurt
- 1 tablespoon homemade tomato puree
- 1 tablespoon fresh lemon juice
- 3-4 garlic cloves, minced
- 2 tablespoons fresh rosemary, chopped
- 2 teaspoons ground coriander
- 1 teaspoon ground cumin
- 1 teaspoon ground cinnamon
- 1 teaspoon red pepper flakes, crushed
- ¼ teaspoon sweet paprika
- Sea salt and freshly ground black pepper, as required
- 1 (4½-pound) bone-in leg of lamb

Directions:

1. In a large bowl, add yogurt, tomato puree, lemon juice, garlic, rosemary, and spices and mix until well combined.
2. Add leg of lamb and coat with marinade generously.
3. Cover and refrigerate to marinate for about 8-10 hours, flipping occasionally.
4. Remove the marinated leg of lamb from refrigerator and keep in room temperature for about 25-30 minutes before roasting.
5. Preheat the oven to 425 degree F.
6. Line a large roasting pan with a greased foil piece.
7. Arrange the leg of lamb into prepared roasting pan.
8. Roast for 20 minutes.
9. Remove the roasting pan from oven and change the side of leg of lamb.
10. Now, Now, reduce the temperature of oven to 325 degree F.
11. Roast for 40 minutes.

12. Now loosely cover the roasting pan with a large piece of foil.
13. Roast for 40 minutes more.
14. Remove from oven and place onto a cutting board for about 10-15 minutes before slicing.
15. With a sharp knife cut the leg of lamb in desired sized slices and serve.
16. Meal Prep Tip: Transfer the leg slices onto a wire rack to cool completely. With foil pieces, wrap the leg slices and refrigerate for about 1-2 days. Reheat in the microwave before serving.

Nutrition Info: Calories 478 Total Fat 15.5 g Saturated Fat 6.1 g Cholesterol 226 mg Total Carbs 3.3 g Sugar 1.3 g Fiber 0.9 g Sodium 226 mg Potassium 48 mg Protein 72.3 g

Beef With Barley & Veggies

Servings: 2

Cooking Time: 1 Hour 5 Minutes

Ingredients:

- ¾ cup filtered water
- ¼ cup pearl barley
- 2 teaspoons olive oil
- 7 ounces lean ground beef
- 1 cup fresh mushrooms, sliced
- ¾ cup onion, chopped
- 2 cups frozen green beans
- ¼ cup low-sodium beef broth
- 2 tablespoon fresh parsley, chopped

Directions:

1. In a pan, add water, barley and pinch of salt and bring to a boil over medium heat.

2. Now, reduce the heat to low and simmer, covered for about 30-40 minutes or until all the liquid is absorbed.

3. Remove from heat and set aside.

4. In a skillet, heat oil over medium-high heat and cook beef for about 8-10 minutes.

5. Add the mushroom and onion and cook f or about 6-7 minutes.

6. Add the green beans and cook for about 2-3 minutes.

7. Stir in cooked barley and broth and cook for about 3-5 minutes more.

8. Stir in the parsley and serve hot.

9. Meal Prep Tip: Transfer the beef mixture into a large bowl and set aside to cool. Divide the mixture into 2 containers evenly. Cover the containers and refrigerate for 1-2 days. Reheat in the microwave before serving.

Nutrition Info: Calories 374 Total Fat 11.4 g Saturated Fat 3.1 g Cholesterol 89 mg Total Carbs 32.7g Sugar 1.1 g Fiber 4.2 g Sodium 136 mg Potassium 895 mg Protein 36.6 g

Taco-stuffed Peppers

Servings: 4

Cooking Time: 15 Minutes

Ingredients:

- 1 pound 80/20 ground beef
- 1 tablespoon chili powder
- 2 teaspoons cumin
- 1 teaspoon garlic powder
- 1 teaspoon salt
- ¼ teaspoon ground black pepper
- 1 (10-ounce) can diced tomatoes and green chiles, drained
- 4 medium green bell peppers
- 1 cup shredded Monterey jack cheese, divided

Directions:

1. In a medium skillet over medium heat, brown the ground beef about 7–10 minutes.

When no pink remains, drain the fat from the skillet.

2. Return the skillet to the stovetop and add chili powder, cumin, garlic powder, salt, and black pepper. Add drained can of diced tomatoes and chiles to the skillet. Continue cooking 3–5 minutes.

3. While the mixture is cooking, cut each bell pepper in half. Remove the seeds and white membrane. Spoon the cooked mixture evenly into each bell pepper and top with a ¼ cup cheese. Place stuffed peppers into the air fryer basket.

4. Adjust the temperature to 350°F and set the timer for 15 minutes.

5. When done, peppers will be fork tender and cheese will be browned and bubbling. Serve warm.

Nutrition Info: Calories: 346 Protein: 27.8 G Fiber: 3.5 G Net Carbohydrates: 7.2 G Fat: 19.1 G Sodium: 991 Mg Carbohydrates: 10.7 G Sugar: 4.9 G

Asian Beef Stir-fry

Servings: 4

Cooking Time: 15 Minutes

Ingredients:

- ¾ lb. beef top sirloin steak, boneless

- 1/3 teaspoon red pepper, crushed

- ½ red onion, wedges

- 3 cups napa cabbage, shredded

- 2 cups broccoli florets

- What you will need from the store cupboard:

- 3 oz. buckwheat noodles or multigrain spaghetti

- 2 tablespoons teriyaki sauce

- 3 tablespoons orange marmalade, low-sugar

- 2 tablespoons of water

- 2 teaspoons canola oil

- Cooking spray

Directions:

1. Bring together the teriyaki sauce, red pepper, marmalade, and water in a bowl.
2. Keep aside. Cook the spaghetti according to directions on the pack.
3. In the meantime, apply cooking spray on your skillet. Preheat.
4. Now add the red onion and broccoli to your skillet.
5. Cook covered for 3 minutes.
6. Add the carrots and cook for 3 more minutes.
7. The vegetables should become tender. Take out the vegetables.
8. Now add oil and the beef strips.
9. Cook for 3 minutes until the center is slightly pink.
10. Return the vegetables to your skillet with the cabbage and sauce.
11. Cook, while stirring, for 1 minute.

Nutrition Info: Calories 279, Carbohydrates 30g, Cholesterol 36mg, Fiber 5g, Sugar 0.8g, Protein 25g, Sodium 259mg

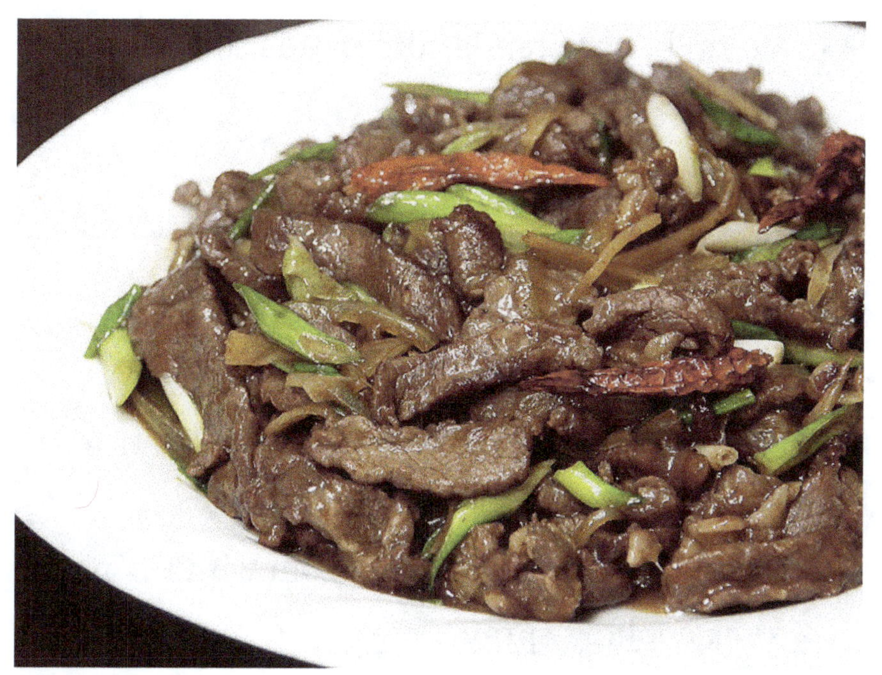

Pork Loin

Servings: 6

Cooking Time: 20 Minutes

Ingredients:

- 1/2 lb. pork tenderloin patted dry
- Non-stick cooking spray
- 2 tbsps. garlic scape pesto
- Salt
- Pepper

Directions:

1. Adjust the temperature of the Air Fryer to 375F.
2. Rub all sides of the tenderloin with the non-stick cooking spray
3. Add pepper, garlic scape pesto, and salt.
4. Sprinkle the Air Fryer basket with cooking spray.
5. Place the tenderloin on the Air Fryer.
6. Cook the meal at 400°F for 10 minutes.

7. Flip over to the other side and cook for another 10 minutes on the first side.

8. Remove the food from the air fryer.

9. Serve

Nutrition Info: Calories: 379 kcal Protein: 8.4g; Fat: 2.2g; Carbs: 0g

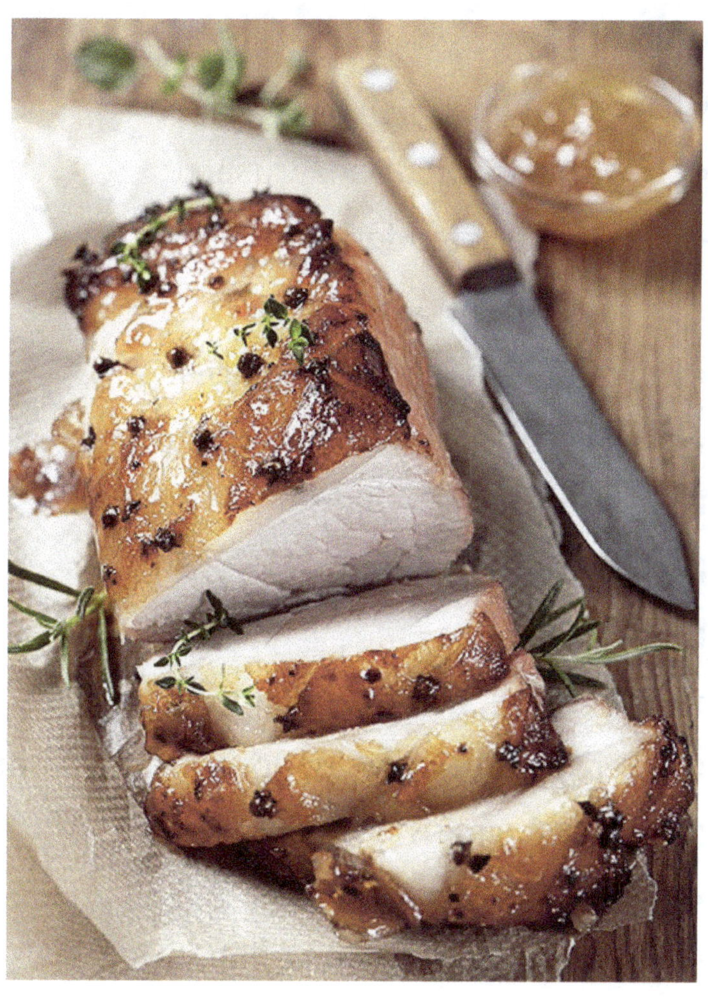

Roasted Pork & Apples

Servings: 4

Cooking Time: 30 Minutes

Ingredients:

- Salt and pepper to taste
- ½ teaspoon dried, crushed
- 1 lb. pork tenderloin
- 1 tablespoon canola oil
- 1 onion, sliced into wedges
- 3 cooking apples, sliced into wedges
- ⅔ cup apple cider
- Sprigs fresh sage

Directions:

1. In a bowl, mix salt, pepper and sage.
2. Season both sides of pork with this mixture.
3. Place a pan over medium heat.
4. Brown both sides.
5. Transfer to a roasting pan.

6.   Add the onion on top and around the pork.

7.   Drizzle oil on top of the pork and apples.

8.   Roast in the oven at 425 degrees F for 10 minutes.

9.   Add the apples, roast for another 15 minutes.

10.   In a pan, boil the apple cider and then simmer for 10 minutes.

11. Pour the apple cider sauce over the pork before serving.

Nutrition Info: Calories 239 Total Fat 6 g Saturated Fat 1 g Cholesterol 74 mg Sodium 209 mg Total Carbohydrate 22 g Dietary Fiber 3 g Total Sugars 16 g Protein 24 g Potassium 655 mg

Nut-stuffed Pork Chops

Servings: 4

Cooking Time: 30 Minutes

Ingredients:

- 3 ounces' goat cheese
- ½ cup chopped walnuts
- ¼ cup toasted chopped almonds
- 1 teaspoon chopped fresh thyme
- 4 center-cut pork chops, butterflied
- Sea salt
- Freshly ground black pepper
- 2 tablespoons olive oil

Directions:

1. Preheat the oven to 400°F.
2. In a small bowl, make the filling by stirring together the goat cheese, walnuts, almonds, and thyme until well mixed.

3. Season the pork chops inside and outside with salt and pepper. Stuff each chop, pushing the filling to the bottom of the cut section. Secure the stuffing with toothpicks through the meat.

4. Place a large skillet over medium-high heat and add the olive oil. Pan sear the pork chops until they're browned on each side, about 10 minutes in total.

5. Transfer the pork chops to a baking dish and roast the chops in the oven until cooked through, about 20 minutes.

6. Serve after removing the toothpicks.

Nutrition Info: Calories: 481 Fat: 38g Protein: 29g Carbs: 5g Fiber: 3g Net Carbs: 2g Fat 70%/Protein 25%/Carbs 5%

Braised Lamb With Vegetables

Servings: 6

Cooking Time: 2 Hours And 15 Minutes

Ingredients:

- Salt and pepper to taste
- 2 ½ lb. boneless lamb leg, trimmed and sliced into cubes
- 1 tablespoon olive oil
- 1 onion, chopped
- 1 carrot, chopped
- 14 oz. canned diced tomatoes
- 1 cup low-sodium beef broth
- 1 tablespoon fresh rosemary, chopped
- 4 cloves garlic, minced
- 1 cup pearl onions
- 1 cup baby turnips, peeled and sliced into wedges
- 1 ½ cups baby carrots
- 1 ½ cups peas

- 2 tablespoons fresh parsley, chopped

Directions:

1. Sprinkle salt and pepper on both sides of the lamb.
2. Pour oil in a deep skillet.
3. Cook the lamb for 6 minutes.
4. Transfer lamb to a plate.
5. Add onion and carrot.
6. Cook for 3 minutes.
7. Stir in the tomatoes, broth, rosemary and garlic.
8. Simmer for 5 minutes.
9. Add the lamb back to the skillet.
10. Reduce heat to low.
11. Simmer for 1 hour and 15 minutes.
12. Add the pearl onion, baby carrot and baby turnips.
13. Simmer for 30 minutes.
14. Add the peas.
15. Cook for 1 minute.
16. Garnish with parsley before serving.

Nutrition Info: Calories 420 Total Fat 14 g Saturated Fat 4 g Cholesterol 126 mg Sodium 529 mg Total Carbohydrate 16 g Dietary Fiber 4 g Total Sugars 7 g Protein 43 g Potassium 988 mg

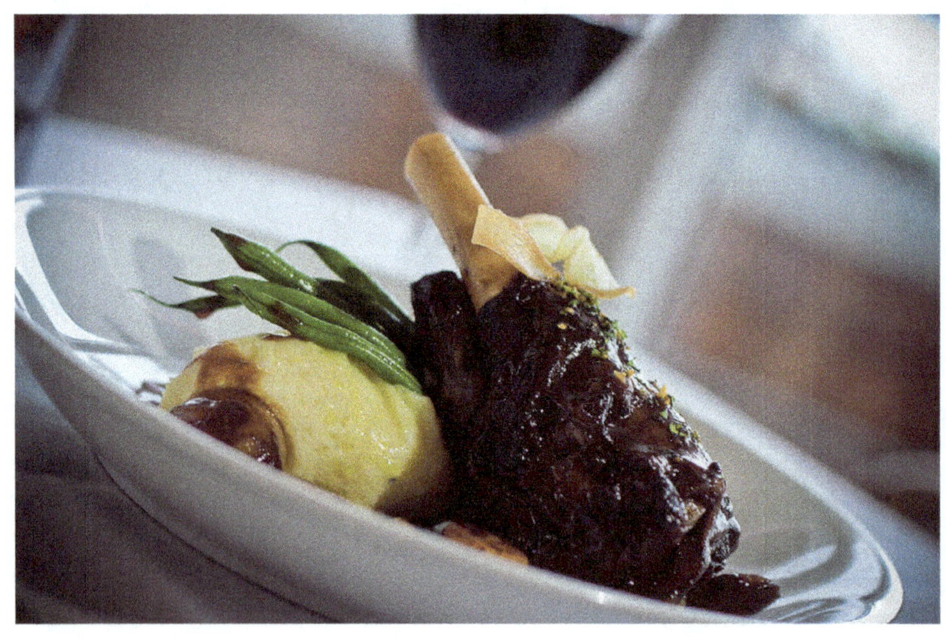

Beef With Broccoli

Servings: 4

Cooking Time: 14 Minutes

Ingredients:

- 2 tablespoons olive oil, divided
- 2 garlic cloves, minced
- 1 pound beef sirloin steak, trimmed and sliced into thin strips
- ¼ cup low-sodium chicken broth
- 2 teaspoons fresh ginger, grated
- 1 tablespoon ground flax seeds
- ½ teaspoon red pepper flakes, crushed
- Salt and ground black pepper, as required
- 1 large carrot, peeled and sliced thinly
- 2 cups broccoli florets
- 1 medium scallion, sliced thinly

Directions:

1. In a large skillet, heat 1 tablespoon of oil over medium-high heat and sauté the garlic for about 1 minute.
2. Add the beef and cook for about 4-5 minutes or until browned.
3. With a slotted spoon, transfer the beef into a bowl.
4. Remove the excess liquid from skillet.
5. In a bowl, add the broth, ginger, flax seeds, red pepper flakes, salt and black pepper.
6. In the same skillet, heat remaining oil over medium heat.
7. Add the carrot, broccoli and ginger mixture and cook for about 3-4 minutes or until desired doneness.
8. Stir in beef and scallion and cook for about 3-4 minutes.
9. Meal Prep Tip: Transfer the beef mixture into a large bowl and set aside to cool. Divide the mixture into 4 containers evenly. Cover

the containers and refrigerate for 1-2 days.
Reheat in the microwave before serving.

Nutrition Info: Calories 211 Total Fat 14.9 g
Saturated Fat 3.9 g Cholesterol 101 mg Total Carbs 6.9
g Sugar 1.9 g Fiber 2.4 g Sodium 108 mg Potassium
706 mg Protein 36.5 g

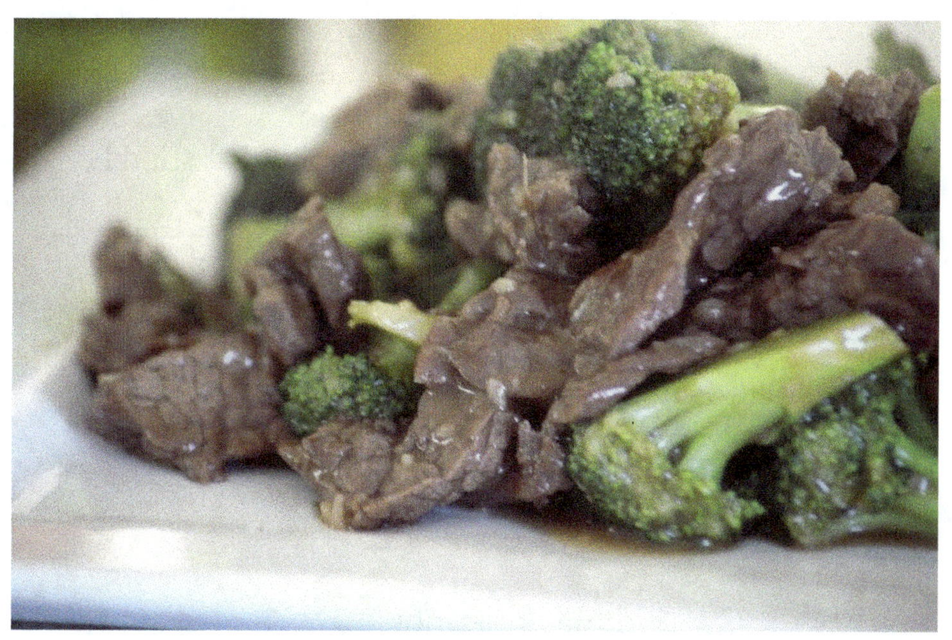

Scrambled Eggs With Sausage

Servings: 2

Cooking Time: 10 Minutes

Ingredients:

- 2 eggs
- ¼ cup cherry tomatoes
- 1 oz. turkey sausage, cooked and sliced
- 1 whole-grain muffin, halved and toasted
- What you will need from the store cupboard:
- 2 tablespoons chicken broth
- 2 tablespoons low-fat Cheddar cheese, shredded
- Ground black pepper
- Cooking spray

Directions:

1. Apply cooking spray on your skillet.
2. Preheat over medium temperature.

3. Whisk together the broth, black pepper and eggs in a bowl.

4. Stir the sliced sausage in.

5. Now pour in the egg mixture.

6. Cook over medium temperature. Don't stir till you see the mixture starting to set around the edges and at the bottom.

7. Lift the fold the egg mix with a spoon or spatula. The uncooked part should flow below.

8. Keep cooking on medium till it is almost set.

9. Now add the cheese and tomatoes.

10. Cook for a minute more.

11. Serve over the toasted muffin halves.

Nutrition Info: Calories 198, Carbohydrates 16g, Fiber 2g, Cholesterol 231mg, Sugar 1g, Fat 9g, Protein 14g

Carnitas

Servings: 2

Cooking Time: 50 Minutes

Ingredients:

- Bay leaves (1)
- Garlic (1 clove slivered)
- Oregano (.25 tsp)
- Garlic powder (.25 tsp)
- Adobo seasoning (.25 tsp.)
- Low-sodium vegetable broth (.25 c)
- Cumin (.5 tsp.)
- Roast (1 lb.)
- Chipotle pepper with adobo sauce (1)

Directions:

1. Set your Instant Pot cooker to sauté.
2. Season the pork as desired before adding it to the Instant Pot cooker and cooking each

side for about 5 minutes. Remove the pork from the pot and set aside to cool.

3.   With the help of a sharp knife, make a 1-in. incision in the pork that is deep enough to accept the garlic slivers.

4.   Add additional seasonings to the pork as desired, rub the mixture into the meat.

5.   Add the broth, bay leaf and the chipotle pepper to the Instant Pot before placing it in the Instant Pot cooker pot and sealing the lid of the cooker. Choose the high-pressure option and set the time for 50 minutes.

6.   Once the timer goes off, select the instant pressure release option and remove the lid. Remove the pork and shred using a pair of forks.

7.   Return the pork to the Instant Pot cooker and allow it to soak up any remaining juices, taking care to remove bay before doing so.

Nutrition Info: Protein: 20 grams Carbs: 12.2 grams Fiber: 11.9 grams Sugar: 11.2 grams Fats: 7.5 grams Calories: 320

Air Fryer Roast Beef

Servings: 3

Cooking Time: 45 Minutes

Ingredients:

- 3-1/2 lbs. beef roast
- 2 tbsps. olive oil
- 1 tbsp. rosemary
- 1/2 tbsp. garlic powder
- 1/2 tsp fresh ground rugged black pepper

Directions:

1. Adjust the temperature of the air fryer to 360°F
2. Mix herbs and oil on a plate. Roll the roast in the blend on the plate to ensure that the entire surface of the beef is covered.
3. Set the beef in the air fryer basket. Establish the timer for 45 mins for tool-rare beef, 51 mins for the tool. Examine the beef with a

meat thermostat to see if it is done to your liking.

4.   Cook for extra 6-minute periods if you like it cooked a lot more. Keep in mind that the roast will undoubtedly remain to prepare while it is relaxing.

5.   Eliminate the roast from the air fryer and put on a plate, cover with lightweight aluminum foil. Allow it to rest for 10 minutes before serving.

Nutrition Info: Calories: 666 kcal; Carbs: 0.3g; Fat: 54g; Proteins: 43g

Pork Chops With Grape Sauce

Servings: 4

Cooking Time: 25 Minutes

Ingredients:

- Cooking spray
- 4 pork chops
- ¼ cup onion, sliced
- 1 clove garlic, minced
- ½ cup low-sodium chicken broth
- ¾ cup apple juice
- 1 tablespoon cornstarch
- 1 tablespoon balsamic vinegar
- 1 teaspoon honey
- 1 cup seedless red grapes, sliced in half

Directions:

1. Spray oil on your pan.
2. Put it over medium heat.
3. Add the pork chops to the pan.

4. Cook for 5 minutes per side.

5. Remove and set aside.

6. Add onion and garlic.

7. Cook for 2 minutes.

8. Pour in the broth and apple juice.

9. Bring to a boil.

10. Reduce heat to simmer.

11. Put the pork chops back to the skillet.

12. Simmer for 4 minutes.

13. In a bowl, mix the cornstarch, vinegar and honey.

14. Add to the pan.

15. Cook until the sauce has thickened.

16. Add the grapes.

17. Pour sauce over the pork chops before serving.

Nutrition Info: Calories 188 Total Fat 4 g Saturated Fat 1 g Cholesterol 47 mg Sodium 117 mg Total Carbohydrate 18 g Dietary Fiber 1 g Total Sugars 13 g Protein 19 g Potassium 759 mg

Pork Roast

Servings: 2

Cooking Time: 3 Hours

Ingredients:

- Coconut oil (1 T)
- Water (2 c)
- Portobello mushrooms (5 sliced thin)
- Garlic (2 cloves smashed)
- Onion (.5 chopped)
- Celery (1 rib)
- Pepper (.5 tsp.)
- Pork roast (1 lb.)

Directions:

1. Start by adding the garlic onion and celery to the Instant Pot cooker pot before adding in the water and then the roast, before seasoning as desired.

2. Place the Instant Pot cooker pot into the
    Instant Pot cooker and seal the lid. Choose
    the high-pressure option and set the time for
    60 minutes.

3. Once the timer goes off, choose the instant
    pressure release option

4. Set the roast aside and place the vegetables
    and resulting broth into a blender and blend
    well.

5. Place the roast back in the Instant Pot
    cooker, seal the cooker and allow it to cook
    for 2 hours under high pressure, this will help
    to render the fat and ensure the edges are
    crisp.

6. When the timer goes off, use the instant
    pressure release option and transfer the roast
    to a serving dish.

7. Turn the Instant Pot cooker to the sauté
    setting before adding in the coconut oil. Once
    it is heated, add in the mushrooms and allow
    them to cook for 5 minutes. Add in the gravy

from the blender and let it reduce until
desired thickness is achieved.

8.   Top roast with gravy prior to serving.

Nutrition Info: Protein: 23.8 grams Carbs: 13.2 grams Fiber: 9 grams Sugar: 2.2 grams Fats: 3.5 grams Calories: 360

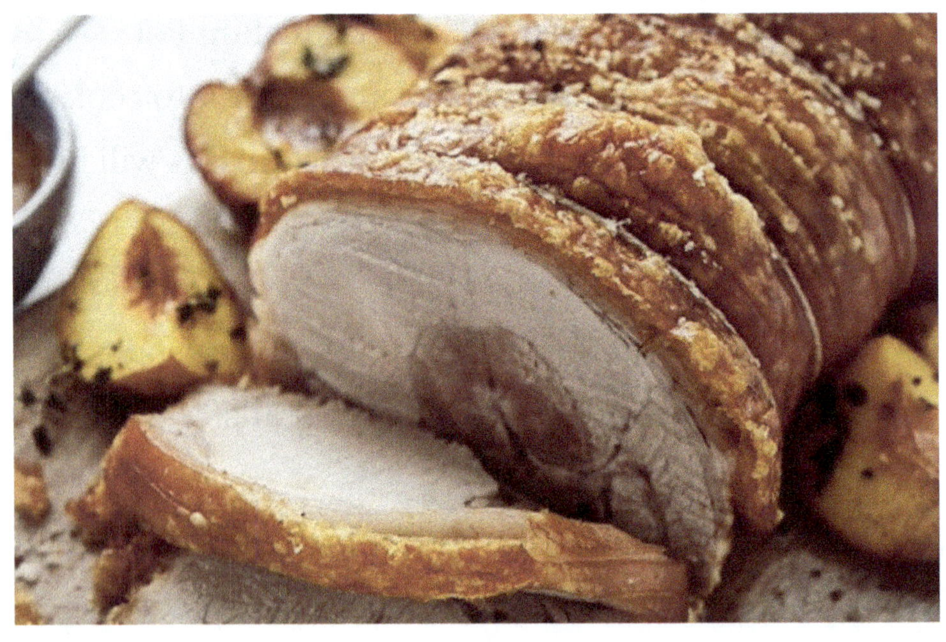

Provencal Ribs

Servings: 4

Cooking Time: 20 Minutes

Ingredients:

- 500g of pork ribs
- Provencal herbs
- Salt
- Ground pepper
- Oil

Directions:

1. Put the ribs in a bowl and add some oil, Provencal herbs, salt, and ground pepper.
2. Stir well and leave in the fridge for at least 1 hour.
3. Put the ribs in the basket of the air fryer and select 2000C for 20 minutes.
4. From time to time, shake the basket and remove the ribs.

Asparagus Beef Sauté

Servings: 4

Cooking Time: 15 Minutes

Ingredients:

- 1 lb. beef tenderloin or sirloin, trimmed and sliced
- 12 oz. asparagus
- 1 carrot, peeled and shredded
- 1 teaspoon crushed herbes de Provence
- ¼ teaspoon lemon peel, grated
- What you will need from the store cupboard:
- ½ cup marsala wine
- 2 teaspoons olive oil
- Cooked rice
- Salt and pepper to taste

Directions:

1. Snap off the asparagus stem ends. Cut into 2-inch pieces.
2. Heat oil over the medium temperature in your skillet.
3. Now cook the carrot, beef, pepper, and salt for 3 minutes. Keep stirring.
4. Add the herbes de Provence and asparagus. Cook for 2 more minutes.
5. Add the lemon peel and marsala. Bring down the heat.
6. Cook for 5 minutes uncovered.
7. Serve with cooked rice.

Nutrition Info: Calories 327, Carbohydrates 29g, Fiber 2g, Cholesterol 69mg, Fat 7g, Sugar 0.3g, Protein 28g, Sodium 209mg

Lamb Leg With Sun-dried Tomato Pesto

Servings: 8

Cooking Time: 70 Minutes

Ingredients:

- FOR THE PESTO
- 1 cup sun-dried tomatoes packed in oil, drained
- ¼ cup pine nuts
- 2 tablespoons extra-virgin olive oil
- 2 tablespoons chopped fresh basil
- 2 teaspoons minced garlic
- FOR THE LAMB LEG
- 1 (2-pound) lamb leg
- Sea salt
- Freshly ground black pepper
- 2 tablespoons olive oil

Directions:

1. TO MAKE THE PESTO

2.   Place the sun-dried tomatoes, pine nuts, olive oil, basil, and garlic in a blender or food processor; process until smooth.

3.   Set aside until needed.

4.   TO MAKE THE LAMB LEG

5.   Preheat the oven to 400°F.

6.   Season the lamb leg all over with salt and pepper.

7.   Place a large ovenproof skillet over medium-high heat and add the olive oil.

8.   Sear the lamb on all sides until nicely browned, about 6 minutes in total.

9.   Spread the sun-dried tomato pesto all over the lamb and place the lamb on a baking sheet. Roast until the meat reaches your desired doneness, about 1 hour for medium.

10.   Let the lamb rest for 10 minutes before slicing and serving.

Nutrition Info: Calories: 352 Fat: 29g Protein: 17g Carbs: 5g Fiber: 2g; Net Carbs: 3g Fat 74%/Protein 20%/Carbs 6%

Ground Pork With Spinach

Servings: 4

Cooking Time: 15 Minutes

Ingredients:

- 1 tablespoon olive oil
- ½ of white onion, chopped
- 2 garlic cloves, chopped finely
- 1 jalapeño pepper, chopped finely
- 1 pound lean ground pork
- 1 teaspoon ground coriander
- 1 teaspoon ground cumin
- ½ teaspoon ground turmeric
- ½ teaspoon ground cinnamon
- ½ teaspoon ground fennel seeds
- Salt and ground black pepper, as required
- ½ cup fresh cherry tomatoes, quartered
- 1¼ pounds collard greens leaves, stemmed and chopped

- 1 teaspoon fresh lemon juice

Directions:

1. In a large skillet, heat the oil over medium heat and sauté the onion for about 4 minutes.

2. Add the garlic and jalapeño pepper and sauté for about 1 minute.

3. Add the pork and spices and cook for about 6 minutes breaking into pieces with the spoon.

4. Stir in the tomatoes and greens and cook, stirring gently for about 4 minutes.

5. Stir in the lemon juice and remove from heat.

6. Serve hot.

7. Meal Prep Tip: Transfer the pork mixture into a large bowl and set aside to cool. Divide the mixture into 4 containers evenly. Cover the containers and refrigerate for 1-2 days. Reheat in the microwave before serving.

Nutrition Info: Calories 316 Total Fat 21.8 g Saturated Fat 0.5 g Cholesterol 0 mg Total Carbs 11.4 g Sugar 1.4 g Fiber 5.7 g Sodium 27 mg Potassium 107 mg Protein 23 g

Vegetable And Egg Muffins

Servings: 6

Cooking Time: 20 Minutes

Ingredients:

- 1 tomato, cored, seeded, and chopped
- 2 teaspoons oregano or rosemary, snipped
- ¼ cup onion, chopped
- ¾ cup zucchini, chopped
- 8 eggs
- What you will need from the store cupboard:
- 1 tablespoon olive oil
- ½ cup crumbled feta cheese
- ⅓ cup bulgur
- ⅔ cup of water
- ⅛ teaspoon black pepper, ground
- Cooking spray

Directions:

1. Preheat your oven to 350 °F.
2. Apply cooking spray to the muffin cups. Keep aside.
3. Combine bulgur and water in a saucepan. Boil and then reduce heat.
4. Simmer until the bulgur becomes tender. Drain off the liquid.
5. Cook the onion and zucchini in your skillet over medium temperature.
6. Remove from heat. Stir the cheese, tomato, and bulgur in.
7. Now spoon the mixture into the muffin cups.
8. Whisk together the pepper, oregano, and eggs in a bowl.
9. Pour the vegetable mix in your muffin cups evenly.
10. Bake for 10-12 minutes.
11. Run a knife around the muffin edges to loosen.
12. Remove muffins carefully from the pans. Serve warm.

Nutrition Info: Calories 117, Carbohydrates 9g, Fiber 2g, Cholesterol 3mg, Sugar 3g, Protein 11g, Sodium 294mg

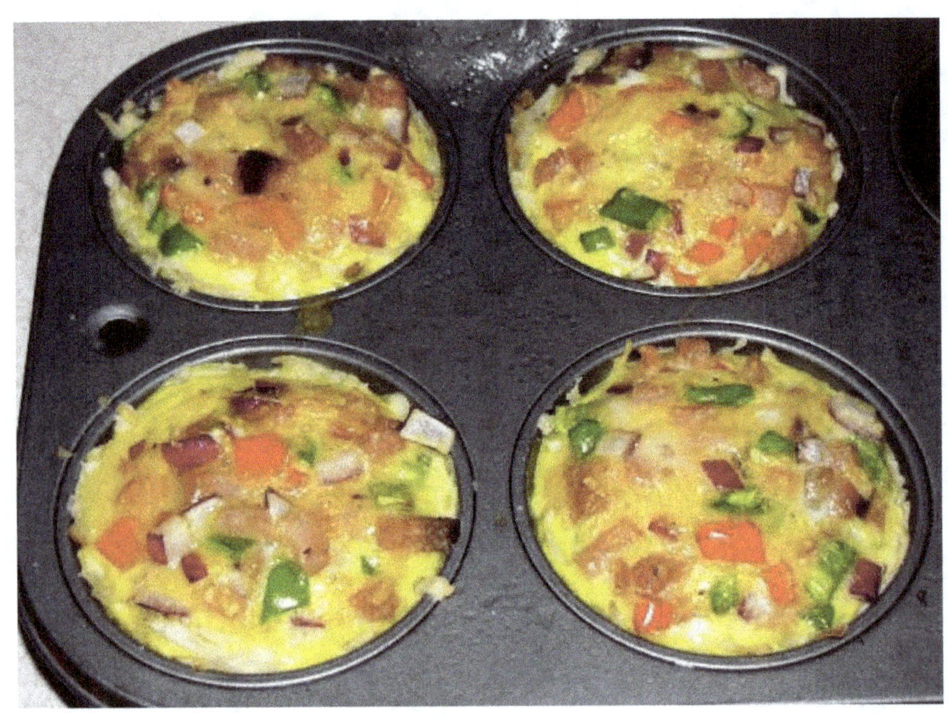

Pork With Bell Peppers

Servings: 4

Cooking Time: 13 Minutes

Ingredients:

- 1 tablespoon fresh ginger, chopped finely
- 4 garlic cloves, chopped finely
- 1 cup fresh cilantro, chopped and divided
- ¼ cup plus 1 tablespoon olive oil, divided
- 1 pound tender pork, trimmed, sliced thinly
- 2 onions, sliced thinly
- 1 green bell pepper, seeded and sliced thinly
- 1 red bell pepper, seeded and sliced thinly
- 1 tablespoon fresh lime juice

Directions:

1. In a large bowl, mix together ginger, garlic, ½ cup of cilantro and ¼ cup of oil.
2. Add the pork and coat with mixture generously.

3. Refrigerate to marinate for about 2 hours.

4. Heat a large skillet over medium-high heat and stir fry the pork mixture for about 4-5 minutes.

5. Transfer the pork into a bowl.

6. In the same skillet, heat remaining oil over medium heat and sauté the onion for about 3 minutes.

7. Stir in the bell pepper and stir fry for about 3 minutes.

8. Stir in the pork, lime juice and remaining cilantro and cook for about 2 minutes.

9. Serve hot.

10. Meal Prep Tip: Transfer the pork mixture into a large bowl and set aside to cool. Divide the mixture into 4 containers evenly. Cover the containers and refrigerate for 1-2 days. Reheat in the microwave before serving.

Nutrition Info: Calories 360 Total Fat 21.8 g Saturated Fat 3.9 g Cholesterol 83 mg Total Carbs 11 g Sugar 5.4 g Fiber 2.2 g Sodium 71 mg Potassium 706 mg Protein 31.2 g

Root Beer Pork

Servings: 2

Cooking Time: 35 Minutes

Ingredients:

- Pork roast (1 lb.)
- Black pepper (as desired)
- Onion (.6 c sliced)
- Root beet (.3 c)
- Ketchup (2 T)
- Almond flour (1.5 tsp)
- Lemon juice (.25 tsp) / Worcestershire sauce (1.5 tsp)
- Tomato paste (1 T) / Honey (1.5 tsp)

Directions:

1. Season roast with pepper and garlic salt, and put in the pot.
2. Mix the rest of the ingredients together and pour on the roast.

3. Lock and seal the lid.

4. Set to meat/stew for 35 minutes. Carefully release pressure

5. Take out onions and roast.

6. Discard the onions and shred the pork.

7. Stir the pork back into the pot.

Nutrition Info: Protein: 19.7grams Carbs: 26.2 grams Fiber: 21.5 grams Sugar: 0 grams Fats: 17.2 grams Calories: 323

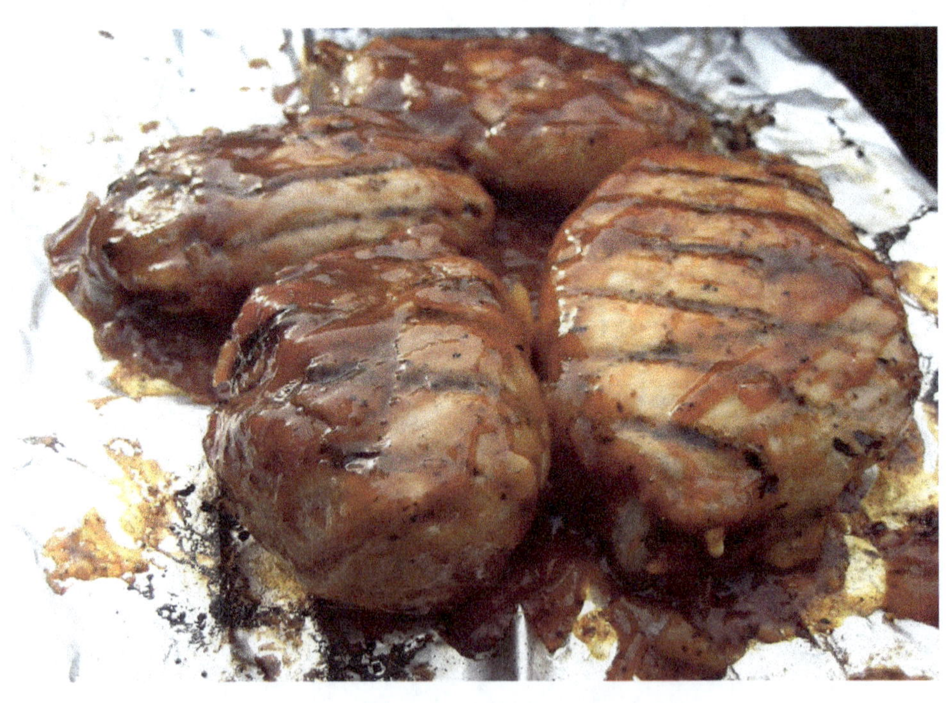

Beef Mushroom Meatballs

Servings: 24 Meatballs

Cooking Time: 30 Minutes

Ingredients:

- 1 tablespoon canola or safflower oil
- 1 (8-ounce) container Portobello mushrooms, finely chopped
- Cooking spray
- 1-pound lean ground beef (90% or higher)
- ¾ cup unseasoned bread crumbs
- ½ cup chopped fresh parsley
- 2 garlic cloves, minced
- 1 egg, beaten
- ¼ teaspoon salt
- ⅛ teaspoon freshly ground black pepper

Directions:

1. In a medium skillet over medium heat, heat the oil until it shimmers. Add the

mushrooms and sauté until they soften, about 5 minutes. Set aside to slightly cool for 5 minutes.

2. Preheat the oven to 350°F. Coat a mini muffin tin with the cooking spray.

3. In a large bowl, combine the mushrooms, beef, bread crumbs, parsley, garlic, egg, salt, and black pepper. Using clean hands, mix until well combined.

4. Form 1 heaping teaspoon of the beef mixture into a 2-inch ball. Place it into a muffin cup and continue forming meatballs.

5. Bake until the meatballs are golden brown, about 25 minutes. Let cool for 5 minutes, then use a teaspoon to transfer each meatball into a storage container.

6. REFRIGERATE: Store the cooled meatballs in a resealable container for up to 1 week. To reheat, microwave for 1 minute. The meatballs also can be reheated in a saucepan over medium heat along with the Speedy Tomato Sauce.

7. FREEZE: Store the cooled meatballs in a freezer-safe container for up to 2 months. Thaw in the refrigerator overnight and reheat in the microwave for 1 minute. The meatballs also can be reheated in a saucepan over medium heat along with the Speedy Tomato Sauce.

Nutrition Info: Calories: 232 Fat: 12g Saturated Fat: 4g Protein: 19g Total Carbs: 12g Fiber: 1g Sodium: 276mg